How's That!

A Layman's Guide to Cricket

Tony Whelpton

with illustrations by

Tim Parker

Published in 2013 by FeedARead.com Publishing
– Arts Council funded

Copyright © Tony Whelpton 1998 and 2013

First Edition

The author has asserted his moral right under the
Copyright, Designs and Patents Act, 1988,
to be identified as the author of this work.

All Rights reserved. No part of this publication may be reproduced,
copied, stored in a retrieval system,
or transmitted, in any form or by any means,
without the prior written consent of the copyright holder,
nor be otherwise circulated in any form of binding or cover
other than that in which it is published and without a similar condition being
imposed on the subsequent purchaser.

A CIP catalogue record for this title is available
from the British Library.

Chapter 1 – Introduction

Why do some people think cricket is a boring game? Because they don't understand it, and, probably, they can't be bothered to try to understand it either. Ask most Englishmen what they think of American football, and they'll say it's slow and boring, because the longest burst of activity in the game lasts for little more than ten seconds, after which there is a break in play which lasts on average about five minutes; compared with that scenario, cricket is the most exciting game on earth! An American would say that just shows they don't understand what's happening. People are the same the world over: if they don't understand something, they'll say it's boring, which is both a confession of their own limitations and an excuse for not bothering to try.

But cricket enthusiasts don't do much to help. Very few of them, if asked, are able to explain, quickly and succinctly, how the game works. Some will say things like 'Cricket is very complicated… It's a way of life… You have to grow up with it…' Others – and this is the problem with most of the books I've seen that have attempted to deal with this – confuse the issue by giving long, technical explanations, with the result that the reader is totally baffled, unable to see the wood for the trees. What is even worse, in their efforts to leaven their over-complicated explanations with humour, they often stray over the border which lies between humour and facetiousness, and they end up belittling the game they profess to love, by making it appear ridiculous.

But cricket is essentially a simple game, and needs to be explained as such. But because it's a very old game, over the years it has become much more sophisticated, and has developed a whole host of subtleties, along with its own jargon, and, of course, it's necessary to understand some of those if one is to get full enjoyment from the modern game.

I've tried to keep the explanations fairly simple, but sometimes a term is used, or a topic is mentioned, which needs fuller treatment if you're to understand the game properly. That's why, at the end of each chapter, you'll find a series of what I've called *Diversions*, which you can either follow at once or leave till later, as you wish. Don't worry about the diversions. They're not more difficult to understand than the rest; it's just that to incorporate them into the main text would make it all unnecessarily complicated, and that's what I want to avoid at all costs. For the same reason, I've relegated a lot of definitions to the *Glossary*, which you'll find at the very end of the book.

Don't think, however, that once you've read this book – diversions included – you'll know all there is to know about cricket, because you won't. This is meant as an introduction to the game, and is written in the hope that you'll not only have a better understanding of what you see, but will want to know and appreciate even more beyond that.

You'll also find that cricket as played on the village green, in public parks, or between local clubs, is rather less subtle than the game I describe, which is essentially the professional game you'll see on television.

Once you've started to understand the game, there's no guarantee that you won't sometimes be bored, whether you understand what's going on or not, because at times the game is played badly, or in the wrong spirit, or the weather ruins any chance of a decisive result. But if that happens, blame the players or the weather by all means, but please don't blame the game!

My thanks are due first of all to a large number of foreign students who, over a period of about fifteen years, used to board with us while studying at a local School of English. They invariably wanted to know why I was spending so many hours watching this strange game on television. It was then that I realised just how difficult it was to explain the game to the layman, and how inadequate all the books in existence were; the obvious answer was to write my own book, and to try it out on these guinea-pigs – from Spain, Italy, Taiwan, Japan, Russia and pretty well any other country you could name – as it progressed. So a special word of thanks to a Spanish boy named Francisco, who eventually started watching cricket on television when I wasn't even in the house!

I also owe an enormous debt of gratitude to the cricketers I have watched over the last sixty-seven years or so, Hammond, Bradman, Lindwall, Hutton, Compton,Graveney, Walsh - the list goes on!

My thanks are also due to Jonathan Agnew and Chris Cowdrey of the BBC Radio 4 *Test Match Special* team, who were kind enough to discuss on air my suggested definition of a 'good length', and who were even kinder in confirming it as accurate. I have only ever been aware of one occasion when Jonathan Agnew has been inaccurate: when he prefaced his remarks about that matter with the words, 'Tony Whelpton is mowing his lawn in Cheltenham at the moment...', when in actual fact I was on my hands and knees trying to mend the wretched lawn-mower which had broken down a moment or two before! I hope that anyone who reads this book and starts to enjoy cricket as a result will quickly come to realise that *Test Match Special* is almost as integral a part of the game as anything I have described in the book!

This book was first published in 1998, and was extremely popular, but it went out of print in 2008 when the original publishers, TD Publications, ceased trading. I decided to publish it as an e-book on the Amazon Kindle Store in 2012, and was overwhelmed by its continued popularity; finally, when I saw that it had reached the number one spot in cricket books in the Kindle Store (practical guides, that is) in both July and August 2013, I decided it was time to re-publish it in paperback form, and that is what you are reading now.

Tony Whelpton
Cheltenham, 1998 and 2013

Chapter 2 – What's it all about?

Cricket is a team game, although, as in baseball, not all members of the team are active at the same time. Sometimes the opposing teams wear different colours, sometimes all the players wear white. Imagine the confusion there would be on a football or a rugby field if all the players wore white! But in cricket it doesn't matter, because it's always clear which side is which: one side is batting and the other side is fielding.

In its simplest, most primitive form, cricket is very straightforward. One player throws a *ball*, another tries to hit it with a piece of wood called a *bat*. There are various ways of deciding how long this goes on for, and also a way of deciding how well the batsman has done. When all the batsmen on one side have had a go, then it's the other side's turn, and the side with the highest score wins the game.

Of course it's a lot more complicated than that really. For the time being we'll forget the matter of scoring and how to tell who's winning, and concentrate on batting and bowling.

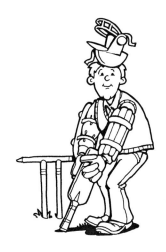

The bowler is the man who throws the ball for the batsman to hit. Except that he doesn't actually *throw* it, because throwing isn't allowed. He *bowls* it, propelling the ball towards the batsman from somewhere up above his head. What's the difference? Well, you *throw* a ball with a bent arm which then straightens, but when you *bowl* a ball the way you do in cricket, your arm is either straight all the time or bent all the time. And also, although I just said that the bowler is the man who throws the ball for the batsman to hit, there's quite a good chance that he would prefer it if the batsman didn't manage to hit it.

What's it all about?

You'll notice that the ball nearly always bounces before it reaches the batsman. This is one of the things that makes cricket more difficult to play than baseball, where the ball comes towards you through the air, without bouncing. Why is it more difficult? Because you can never be quite sure what the ball is going to do after it bounces, and it bounces so close to you that you don't have much time in which to react.

That's why you often see people bowling slowly. If a baseball pitcher threw the ball slowly, it would just make it easier to hit, but in cricket a slow bowler usually spins the ball, either by using his fingers or turning his wrist, and that means it will probably change direction when it bounces. The trouble is you don't always know which way it will turn – towards you or away from you. Moreover, you don't know how high it will bounce either, or whether it will speed up once it has pitched. It might even slow down, which could mean that you play your shot too early and then miss the ball altogether.

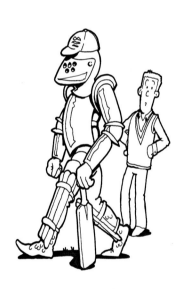

You'll understand why batsmen wear protective helmets!

Sometimes, though, you see a fast bowler in action, and when I say fast I mean the ball comes towards you very fast – anything up to 90 or 100 miles an hour (150 or 160 kph). And when I tell you that some of those bowlers can make the ball change direction, either while it's in the air or after it bounces – and sometimes both! – and that a ball bouncing six feet in front of you can suddenly come shooting up towards your head (and a cricket ball is harder than a baseball!) then you'll understand why batsmen wear protective helmets! Of course if the ball bounced like that every time, it would make the game easier, but it doesn't – it sometimes stays low, even when it appears to have bounced in exactly the same place as the one that nearly took your head off a couple of minutes ago!

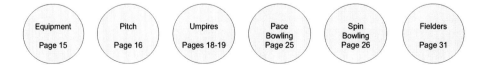

Equipment	Pitch	Umpires	Pace Bowling	Spin Bowling	Fielders
Page 15	Page 16	Pages 18-19	Page 25	Page 26	Page 31

You'll notice that I've rather sneakily put you in the position of being the batsman. So what do you do when you see this ball coming towards you? Well, you either hit it or miss it. But if you miss it, you may have missed it accidentally or on purpose.

And if you hit it, you may have hit it hard, or you may have hit it gently. It depends what you're trying to do; in fact, it's the classic choice you have in most games, the choice between attack and defence, or, put another way, a matter of playing the percentages, or choosing the option which gives you the best chance of success.

You'll notice that the batsman doesn't often hit across the ball like a baseball player does. That's because, over a period of many years – hundreds of them! – it has been found that the most effective way of dealing with a ball whose bounce is extremely unpredictable, and whose trajectory can be deceptive, is to play with a straight bat, that is with the bat at more or less right angles to the ground. That's sometimes referred to as 'playing down the line'.

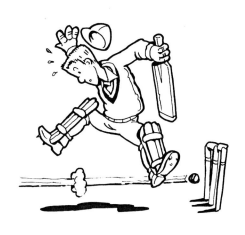

What do you do when you see this ball coming towards you?

So where have we got to? We've got the bowler bowling the ball, and the batsman hitting it – or not, as the case may be. Now we come to a very important matter: how do you decide how long a batsman bats? Well, have a look behind the batsman, and you'll see three upright pieces of wood (called *stumps*), with two little pieces of wood (called *bails*) balanced on top. This is called the *wicket*, and if the bowler manages to hit the wicket with the ball, the batsman is *out*, and his *innings* is over.

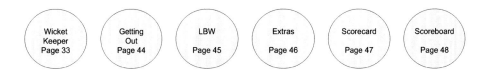

Wicket
Keeper
Page 33

Getting
Out
Page 44

LBW

Page 45

Extras

Page 46

Scorecard

Page 47

Scoreboard

Page 48

But that isn't the only way of getting him out. If the batsman hits the ball, and then it's caught by one of the other side – without bouncing, that is – then that's out too. And if he stops the ball hitting his wicket by putting his leg (or any other part of his body) in the way, that can be out as well, although the rules on that are a bit complicated and I'll explain those later. There are one or two other ways of getting out, but we can safely leave those till later too.

So part of the batsman's job is to avoid getting out – but, unlike the batsman in the cartoon, he's not allowed to do that by using a huge bat!

As long as he's not out he can go on batting as long as he likes (at least, within reason – there are limits!). But he also has to make a contribution to his team's score, and he does that by hitting the ball hard enough to make *runs*.

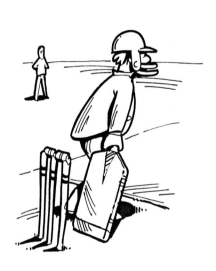

The batsman's job is to avoid getting out...

To score one run, the batsman must run to the bowler's end of the pitch (which, incidentally, is 22 yards long). To score a second run, he must run back again. In other words, for each length of the pitch he runs, he scores one run.

Sometimes the batsman hits the ball so hard it goes right to the edge of the field, known as the *boundary*; if he does, he scores four runs. If he manages to hit the ball over the boundary without bouncing, he scores six.

Now you're probably thinking – if he scores one run by running to the bowler's end, he's in the wrong place the next time the bowler runs in to bowl, so what does he do? After all, it would be a waste of time if he had to walk back to his place every time.

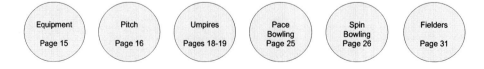

Equipment	Pitch	Umpires	Pace Bowling	Spin Bowling	Fielders
Page 15	Page 16	Pages 18-19	Page 25	Page 26	Page 31

The answer is that there are always two batsmen in at the same time, and they both have to run the length of the pitch for a run to be added to the score; that ensures that there will always be a batsman in the right place, ready to receive the next ball. It also adds to the excitement, because another way of getting the batsman out is for the bowling side to hit the wicket with the ball before the run is completed. If there are two batsmen, the chances of that happening are increased, especially since you find that misunderstandings between the two batsmen sometimes result in one of them running and the other staying put!

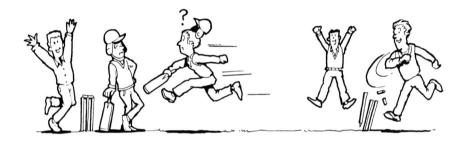

Misunderstandings sometimes occur...

You'll have realised, I'm sure, that there will eventually come a time when there is no one left to come in, and yet one batsman is still there – not out. And that's how it will stay – the innings is over – because there must *always* be two batsmen in at the same time. When that point is reached, we say the side is *all out*.

Let's go back to the bowler for a moment. Bowling, especially bowling fast, is an extremely energetic activity, and to do it effectively you need to do it in short bursts. What actually happens is that a bowler is only allowed to bowl six balls in succession, and then someone else takes over, bowling the next six balls from the other end of the pitch. And because someone else is taking *over*, each series of six balls is called an *over*. That enables a bowler to carry on bowling for quite a long time – perhaps even seven or eight overs in succession, which would be impossible if they didn't have a break in between.

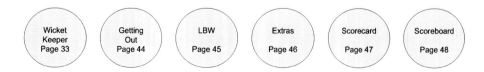

Wicket Keeper Page 33 — Getting Out Page 44 — LBW Page 45 — Extras Page 46 — Scorecard Page 47 — Scoreboard Page 48

Now let's go back to the start of the game. The two captains toss a coin to decide which team will bat first. The one who wins the toss may decide to bat, or he may ask the other side to bat first. His decision will be based on a whole host of other factors – whether the pitch looks easy to bat on, the relative strength of the teams, and, in particular, the weather, which can have a great effect on the outcome of a match.

Once the batting side begin their innings, they carry on batting until they're all out, or until their captain decides they've batted long enough, and stand a good chance of winning even if they don't score any more runs.

Then the other side goes in and, in the simplest form of the game, they bat until they're all out without passing the other side's score (in which case they've lost), or until they've passed that score (in which case they've won). If the time allotted to the game is all used up before that point is reached, then the game ends in a *draw*.

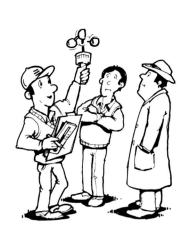

Sometimes, though, a set amount of time is allocated to each innings. Usually, at least in international and other matches played at the top level, each innings is fifty (or sometimes only twenty) overs long. In these cases there is always a winner and a loser. Even if the number of runs scored by each side is the same, there will be some way of deciding which side has actually won, for instance by looking at the number of wickets they've lost in the course of their allotted overs.

In some games each side is allowed to bat twice, and the runs scored in each innings are added together to decide who's won. This is what happens, for instance, in *test matches* (international matches), which may last up to five days.

His decision may be based on the weather

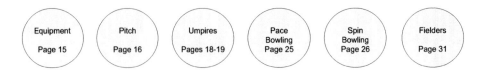

Equipment	Pitch	Umpires	Pace Bowling	Spin Bowling	Fielders
Page 15	Page 16	Pages 18-19	Page 25	Page 26	Page 31

People from countries where little or no cricket is played often express bewilderment at the thought of a match lasting for as long as five days. Some sports, however, can last almost as long, or even longer: a major golf tournament is spread over four days, whilst the *Tour de France* cycle race lasts as long as three weeks!

So far I've only referred specifically to three people who are on the field – the bowler and two batsmen, but in fact there are twelve others. Two of these are there to see that the players don't break the rules and also to judge, when asked, whether a batsman is out or not. They are called the *umpires*, and if a player wants them to make that sort of decision, he *appeals* to them, usually by shouting 'How's that?' They also look after players' sweaters, sun-hats, etc., when they don't need them.

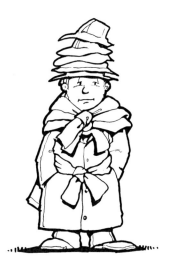

And then, of course, there are the bowler's team-mates, ten in number, placed at different points in the field, and called *fielders*. The fielders basically have three functions:

They also look after players' sweaters and sun-hats

(i)   to retrieve the ball and get it back to the bowler so the game can continue as quickly as possible;
(ii)   to try to stop the batting side scoring runs, or at least restrict the number of runs they score;
(iii)   to help to get the batsman out.

The fielder who is most often in the action is the *wicket-keeper*. He is the one who stands behind the wicket and is the only one to wear gloves. He is the busiest of all because if the batsman misses the ball, whether by accident or design, the ball goes through to the wicket-keeper, and he has to stop it. Also, if the batsman hits the ball and it is picked up by a fielder, the fielder will nearly always throw it back to the wicket-keeper rather than straight back to the bowler.

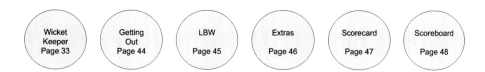

Wicket Keeper Page 33 | Getting Out Page 44 | LBW Page 45 | Extras Page 46 | Scorecard Page 47 | Scoreboard Page 48

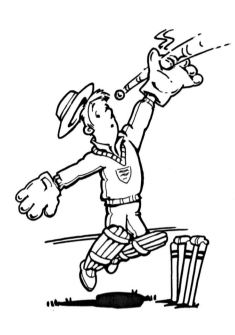

If the batsman misses the ball, the wicket-keeper has to stop it...

Incidentally, if the batsman and the wicket-keeper both miss the ball, the batsmen are allowed to run, thus adding to their team's score. These runs, called *byes*, are added to the team's total, but not to the individual batsman's, and they are just one of a number of ways of scoring runs other than as a result of the batsman hitting the ball. Such runs are called *extras* (or, in Australia, *sundries*).

By now you should have a pretty good idea of what the game is about. In the remaining chapters we'll look more closely at each aspect of the game. The *Diversions* will tell you even more; look at these when you feel the need.

Diversion 1 – Equipment

Clothing: Traditionally, all players wear white, but in recent years coloured clothing has become the norm for the limited-over game.

Boots normally have short spikes in the soles to prevent the players slipping on the grass playing-surface, but if they are wearing spikes they have to be especially careful when running on the pitch because of the damage the spikes can cause to the surface.

Batting gloves are worn by the batsman to protect the fingers.

Wicket-keeping gloves, which are much bigger than batting gloves, usually with webbing between the fingers, are worn by the wicket-keeper to protect his hands. No other fielder wears gloves.

A helmet may be worn by the batsman to protect his head when facing fast bowling, or by a fielder when fielding close to the bat.

Pads are worn by both batsmen and wicket-keeper to protect their legs.

Arm-guards are sometimes worn on a batsman's forearm (the left arm for a right-hander, the right arm for a left-hander) when he is facing fast bowling.

The only other visible items of clothing are likely to be sun-hats or peaked caps, and occasionally sunglasses or light-enhancing glasses. In addition players, especially batsmen, wicket-keepers and close fielders, will wear various kinds of padding to protect shins, thighs, chest, and other vulnerable areas.

The ball is hard, usually red but sometimes white, and encased in leather with a stitched seam around its 9" circumference. It weighs about 5½ ounces.

The bat is made of wood (invariably willow), and is about three feet long. The flat blade (the part used to strike the ball) is just over 4" wide. The handle is normally covered with rubber, and is sprung to absorb the vibrations set up when the ball is struck.

The wicket consists of three round wooden stumps, 28" high, with grooves to house the two wooden bails, which are placed on top. When pitched, the wicket is thus 28½" high and 9" wide.

Equipment
Page 15

Equipment
Page 15

Diversion 2 – The Pitch

First of all a distinction must be made between the *pitch*, the *square*, and the *playing area*. The playing area is the entire area of ground circumscribed by the boundary. The square is an area in the middle of the playing area which is looked after particularly carefully by the groundsman, because a strip from that area will be used as the pitch.

This strip (also sometimes referred to, somewhat confusingly, as the *wicket*) is 10 feet wide and 22 yards long. At the start of the match the grass on the pitch will be cut extremely short, rolled, and the stumps set at either end.

The three wooden *stumps*, surmounted by the *bails*, are set close enough together to stop the ball passing between them, at the centre of a white line known as the *bowling crease*. Four feet in front of the stumps, and parallel to the bowling crease, is another white line known as the *popping crease*. (When the stumps are set, this too is known as the *wicket*. However, any likelihood of confusion is more apparent than real, because the context will always tell you whether the word *wicket* is being used to mean the *stumps* or the *pitch*.)

At each end of the bowling crease, and at right angles to it, another white line is painted. This is called the *return crease*, and the box formed by these four lines is known as the batsman's *ground*. As you will see from the diversion *Ways of getting out*, if a batsman is 'out of his ground', he is in danger of being given out either *run out* or *stumped*. When facing the bowler, therefore, the batsman will stand just inside his ground, with the tip of his bat resting on or near the popping crease.

The condition of the pitch has such an effect on the behaviour of the ball that great efforts are made to ensure that it doesn't become unduly damp (through rain) or damaged (by the spikes in the soles of the players' boots). That is why the players leave the field and the pitch is covered immediately it starts raining, and why bowlers are sometimes warned by the umpires for running on the pitch.

Finally, one side of the pitch is known as the *off side*, the other as the *on side* or the *leg side*. Imagine you are standing behind the stumps at the bowler's end (where the umpire is in the diagram). If the batsman facing you is right-handed, the off side will be to your left, the leg side to your right. If he is left-handed he will be standing on the other side of the wicket, so in that case the off side will be to your right and the leg side to your left.

Pitch
Page 16

Pitch
Page 16

The Pitch

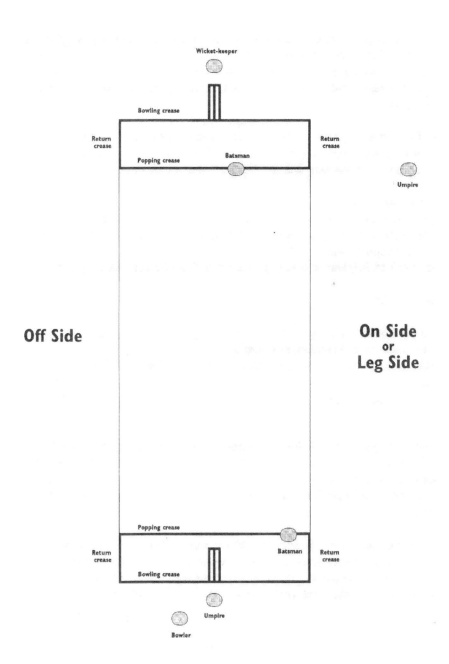

Diversion 3 – The Umpires

There are two umpires (who until recently used to wear white coats, but these days they are dressed more casually – the most important factor being that they must be dressed differently from the players). One stands just behind the stumps at the bowler's end, the other stands at square leg. At the end of each over the umpires reverse positions, the square leg umpire going to the bowler's wicket and vice versa. Although their main function is to ensure that the game is played according to the rules, they have a lot of other responsibilities too.

Before the game, they have to check that the pitch and the weather conditions are fit for play; if they're not satisfied, then the game won't start. Then they have to get the two captains together and toss a coin to decide who will bat first and who will bowl.

During the game they have to

(i) keep count of the number of balls bowled in an over, and call 'over' after each series of six;

(ii) tell the scorers by using hand-signals whether a batsman is out, a boundary has been scored or extras have been scored;

(iii) keep check of the time or the number of overs bowled and make sure play ends at the right time;

(iv) watch the play closely, so they are in a position to give a decision when asked by the fielding side;

(v) watch the bowler carefully to make sure his bowling is within the laws. This includes calling no-balls and wides (See diversion on Extras);

(vi) decide whether to suspend play because of bad weather or bad light;

(vii) keep check of the condition of the ball (although the bowler will usually not be slow to complain if the ball has gone out of shape).

When the fielders appeal for the batsman to be given out (by shouting 'How's that?'), the umpire either says 'Not out' or indicates that he is out by raising his index finger above his head. He indicates a boundary four by waving his arm from side to side and a boundary six by raising both arms above his head. The other important signals he gives are dealt with in the diversion on Extras.

You will also sometimes hear of a Third Umpire. For a definition of his role, see the Diversion headed DRS.

Umpires
Pages 18-19

Umpires
Pages 18-19

Diversion 4 - DRS and the Third Umpire

Sometimes you will hear a reference to a 'third umpire'. The third umpire never comes on to the field of play. Instead, he watches television replays and makes decisions, if asked, on such matters as whether the ball has crossed the boundary, or whether a batsman managed to regain his ground before the wicket was broken in a run-out attempt.

The Third Umpire is also involved in something new (and controversial). It's called D.R.S.

In the first-class game, and especially in international cricket, D.R.S. has become increasingly important. It stands for Decision Review System, and it comes into operation – provided both sides agree that it should be used – when one side or the other is not convinced that an umpire's decision is correct.

Thus, if a batsman is given out caught because the umpire believes he 'edged' the ball to the wicket-keeper, he may call for a review if he is convinced that his bat (or his glove) did not touch the ball. In this case a third umpire (unsurprisingly called 'The Third Umpire') looks at a television replay and either confirms or rescinds the original decision.

Similarly, a bowler who has just had his appeal for *Leg Before Wicket* turned down may request a review, and again the Third Umpire will judge on the basis of a television replay.

In order to prevent the review system getting out of hand, each side is limited to two unsuccessful reviews per innings (that is the team's entire innings, not an individual batsman's innings).

At the time of writing, this system is used in all test matches except those involving India, whose controlling authority is not convinced as to its efficacy or its fairness.

Umpires
Pages 18-19

Umpires
Pages 18-19

Chapter 3 – More about bowling

Cricket is a bit like chess, though admittedly with a lot more action. But behind each action there is a lot of thinking going on, and all is not necessarily as it seems. A team's tactics will vary a good deal, of course, according to whether they're batting or bowling, but they will also vary according to the current state of the match, the weather, the state of the pitch, and also according to what they know or have observed about the other side.

Let's start with the bowler. You might think that because the primary way of getting a batsman out is to *bowl* him by hitting his stumps, that is what the bowler will be trying to do every time, and he will do that by bowling straight. But of course that would be too predictable, and to allow the batsman to predict accurately what you're going to do is one of the worst things you can do if you're a bowler – you have to keep him guessing. In any case, there are a number of other ways of getting a batsman out apart from bowling him.

The early part of a batsman's innings – before he has 'got his eye in' – is the time when he is most vulnerable, and part of the bowler's job is to try and stop him settling into a groove. One way to do that is to get him out, and essentially that's what the bowler would like. But it's unrealistic for a bowler to think he's going to take a wicket with every ball he bowls, and a lot of wickets are taken as a result of the bowler having created some uncertainty in the batsman's mind, probably over a period of time. In other words, it's a battle of wits as much as a battle between bat and ball.

So, what options are open to the bowler if he wants to be unpredictable? First of all there is the matter of *line*. That means the direction in which he bowls. The first decision he must make is whether to bowl *over* or *round* the wicket. For a right-handed bowler, *over the wicket* means that, when he bowls, the wicket at his end is on his right; in other words, his bowling arm is literally 'over the wicket' as he bowls.

A straight ball bowled over the wicket, therefore, unless it turned or swung one way or the other, or bounced too high, would hit the stumps at the other end – always assuming, of course, that the batsman didn't stop it doing so.

If the bowler bowls *round the wicket*, with the stumps to his left, then the angle of delivery has changed, and the batsman will have to take that into account. (Some bowlers, of course, are left-handed, and so *over the wicket* and *round the wicket* for them would be the other way round.)

The *Diversions* dealing with the different types of bowling will give you some idea as to how the direction of the ball can change either before or after it bounces. The good bowler will vary the type of ball he bowls, whilst all the time taking good care to prevent the batsman seeing (for instance, by looking at the way he holds the ball in his hand) that he is going to do something different. Whatever he does, he wants the batsman to be wondering in what direction the ball will be travelling when it reaches him. It goes without saying, of course, that it will be travelling towards him, but when the bat is only 4.25 inches (108 mm) wide and the ball is approaching you at 90 mph (145 kph), a variation of only a fraction of an inch in the ball's trajectory can make a big difference.

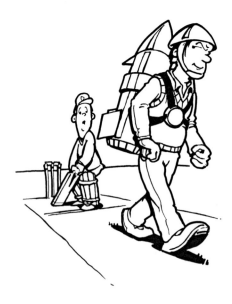

A really fast bowler...

Then there is the matter of *length* – where will the ball bounce? Will it be short, pitched up, or a 'full toss' (which means it doesn't actually bounce at all). We can effectively rule out a full toss because, as I've already said, a ball which doesn't bounce is easier to hit than one that does. And for any but the fastest bowlers, bowling short is a bad idea because again it is easier to hit. This is because when the ball bounces, it rises at first, then starts to fall, and it's easier to hit a falling ball than a rising one. If a really fast bowler pitches the ball short, however, it will still be rising when it reaches the batsman, and that's a lot more difficult to cope with.

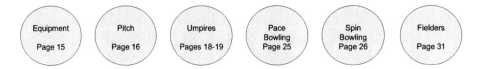

Equipment	Pitch	Umpires	Pace Bowling	Spin Bowling	Fielders
Page 15	Page 16	Pages 18-19	Page 25	Page 26	Page 31

But between 'too short' and 'too long' there are lots of other possibilities, because as with *line*, a few inches longer or shorter can make a lot of difference. One thing that happens is this: if a ball is pitched short, the batsman's instinctive first movement is to step back a little, because that's the most comfortable way of playing short bowling. If it's pitched up, the natural movement is forward. But there's a point somewhere in the middle where the batsman isn't quite sure whether to go forward or back, and such uncertainty can lead to a false shot and possibly the loss of his wicket. A ball that does that is called a *good length ball*.

A further possible variation is that of *pace*. A bowler capable of bowling at 100 mph won't bowl every ball at that speed. Sometimes he will bowl it just a little bit more slowly, preferably without giving the batsman any indication that that's what he's going to do.

The same goes for a *slow bowler*, who will sometimes bowl one ball just a little bit faster than the previous one, again in the hope of creating uncertainty.

A further possibility for the slow bowler is variation in *flight*. Sometimes he may bowl the ball so that it goes quite high before falling a couple of feet or so in front of the batsman. Another time he may bowl it 'flat', without making it go up in the air at all.

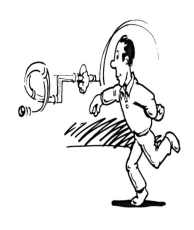

When the ball is 'flighted' in this way it is normally *spinning* – sometimes quite fast – and, depending on the type of spin, the flight will vary. The ball may suddenly dip in its flight, and then shoot forward as it lands, or it may hold back, inducing the batsman to play his shot too early. Once again it's a question of creating uncertainty in the mind of the batsman.

A further possibility for the slow bowler is variation in flight.

| Wicket Keeper Page 33 | Getting Out Page 44 | LBW Page 45 | Extras Page 46 | Scorecard Page 47 | Scoreboard Page 48 |

So far we've assumed that the bowler is trying to get the batsman out. But that isn't always the case. Sometimes he may just want to stop him scoring runs, especially in a *limited-overs* game where the team which scores most in a certain number of overs will win, even if they haven't got the other side all out.

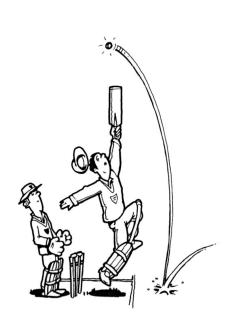

So high that the batsman can't reach it!

Restricting the batsman's scoring opportunities can be a question of field-placing, and I'll deal with that in the next chapter. But some types of delivery are easier than others to score from, so bowlers in such circumstances develop strategies to help them stop the batsman scoring.

One thing they're not allowed to do, though, is bowl the ball so wide, or so high, that the batsman can't reach it! If they do that, it's called a *wide*, and one run is added to the batting side's score. If the wicket-keeper can't reach it either, and it goes to the boundary, then that counts as four wides, and four runs are added to the score, classed as *extras*.

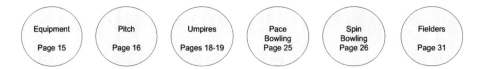

Diversion 5 – Pace Bowling

A genuinely fast bowler can get a batsman out by the sheer speed with which he hurls the ball down; obviously the faster it comes, the less time the batsman has to react. If the batsman misses a straight ball, then of course he's likely to be out bowled or leg before wicket, but in fact fast bowlers probably take more wickets with balls bowled outside the line of the stumps than with straight balls.

That's because the ball comes so fast that the batsman either doesn't have time to pull his bat out of the way, or he tries to hit the ball and mistimes the shot. In either case the ball is likely to hit the edge of the bat rather than the middle, and the ball is then caught by the wicket-keeper or by one of the fielders standing at *slip* or *short-leg*.

Sometimes, though, a bowler who bowls at a slightly slower pace (though still pretty fast) can be more effective, because he is able to make the ball *swing* in the air as it approaches the batsman – sometimes before it bounces, sometimes after. If the ball swings in towards the batsman it's called an *in-swinger*; if it swings the other way it's called an *out-swinger* or an *away-swinger*.

A number of factors affect which way the ball will swing, or whether it will swing at all: the way the bowler holds the ball, the condition of the ball itself, and – the weather! Although some physicists disagree – some to the point of denying that the ball swings at all! – anyone who has ever played cricket knows that on a hot summer's day the ball swings less than when there's a lot of cloud cover and the atmosphere is heavy and humid.

You will often see cricketers polishing the ball – usually on their trousers, to the delight of laundry proprietors! But they only polish one side of the ball, because if one side is more highly polished than the other the air resistance on that side of the ball will be reduced, and that will cause the ball to swing. The same effect could be obtained by roughening up the other side of the ball, but that is illegal, and anyone caught doing it would be branded as a cheat (which for a cricketer would be the ultimate disgrace). The bowler then holds the ball in such a way that the seam is pointing in the direction in which he wants the ball to swing. But he has to hold it the right way round too: if he wants the ball to swing from right to left he must hold the ball so that the shiny side is on the right, and vice versa.

(The *medium-pace* bowler can also sometimes do what a spin bowler does, but a bit faster – to learn more, read the Diversion on Spin bowling.)

Pace Bowling Page 25

Pace Bowling Page 25

Diversion 6 – Spin Bowling

Not all bowlers bowl fast, and very fast bowling is not always the most effective; sometimes slow bowling brings greater rewards. But a slow bowler needs to be more subtle: he needs to be able to *spin* the ball, because, when a spinning ball hits the ground, it changes direction, and the batsman can sometimes be deceived because he's not sure which way the ball is going to turn, or how much it's going to turn. What's more, a bowler will sometimes send one down which doesn't turn at all, and if the batsman is assuming that, because the previous five deliveries have turned so will the sixth, he could be in trouble.

Whether the ball turns or not depends on how the bowler holds it, and how he turns his hand or spins the ball with his fingers at the moment of delivery. For this reason a spin bowler will often try to stop the batsman being able to see how he's holding the ball.

It also depends on the state of the pitch. In a *first-class match*, that is one between, for instance, two English counties, or in a *test match* (an international fixture) the pitches are so well prepared that it's often only in the later stages of the game that the ball will turn when it lands. In club matches, often played in public parks on pitches that are well-worn through constant use, the ball will usually spin much more.

You might think that the answer to this would be for the batsman to move down the pitch towards the bowler and hit the ball before it bounces, thus smothering the spin, and you would be right – up to a point. Unfortunately for the batsman, spin can also affect the flight of the ball, and if he goes forward like that and misses the ball completely, he is likely to be out *stumped* – if you don't understand that, look at the Diversion on Ways of getting out.

When a bowler spins the ball, he may be bowling *leg-breaks* or *off-breaks*. This simply indicates which way the ball will turn when it lands: a leg-break is one which will turn from *the leg-side* towards *the off*, whilst an off-break will turn from *the off-side* towards *the leg*. To confuse the issue – and the batsman! – even more, many bowlers are able to turn the ball one way whilst looking as if they're going to turn it the other. These types of delivery have different names, e.g. *googly*, *Chinaman*, *wrong 'un*, but we don't need to go into the finer details of that here – one could write a whole book on that aspect of bowling alone!

Then there is a top-spinner, which doesn't move from side to side but suddenly speeds up as it lands, and probably bounces higher than the batsman expects.

Spin Bowling Page 26

Spin Bowling Page 26

Chapter 4 – More about fielding

If one objective of the fielding side is to restrict scoring opportunities, then obviously the fielders must be placed in positions where the ball is most likely to be hit. To a certain extent this is determined by the type of bowling. It's unusual, for instance, for a batsman to be able to hit a ball from a fast bowler back high above the bowler's head, so you'll hardly ever see a fielder standing on the boundary behind a fast bowler. With a slow bowler, however, this is more of a possibility, so you will sometimes see a man placed there.

But if another objective is to help to get the batsman out, then the fielders must be placed in positions where they're most likely to be able to do this. That effectively means positions to which the ball is likely to go at catching height. Theoretically, of course, that could mean anywhere, but in reality there are some parts of the field to which the ball is much more likely to go than others, depending upon the type of bowling.

Some fielders have extremely quick reactions, and seem able to catch anything, with either hand, at whatever height, and however fast it's travelling. (What's more, they *never* wear gloves!) It therefore makes sense to put these close to the batsman, because that's where such opportunities arise most frequently. In the modern international game, however, all players are more athletic than used to be the case, and many are capable of fielding anywhere in the field.

Others are particularly good at stopping a ball hit very hard along the ground, and then picking it up and throwing it almost in a single movement. These are the ones who will stand where the ball is most likely to be hit hard, notably *cover*, *point* (or *backward point*), *mid-wicket*, *mid-on* and *mid-off*.

Basically there are two types of field-placing – *offensive* and *defensive*. With an offensive field you'll see more fielders close to the bat and hardly anyone back on the boundary. When a defensive field is set, you'll find hardly anyone close to the bat, and most of them standing well back – perhaps allowing the batsman to score the odd one or two, but trying to limit the number of boundaries scored.

Setting an offensive field puts pressure on the batsman – he sees himself surrounded by men all eager to grab the ball if it flies off the edge of his bat.

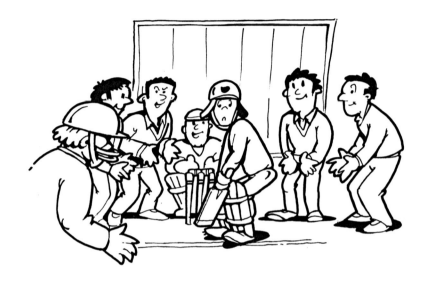

Surrounded by men all eager to grab the ball...

But setting an attacking field also entails a certain risk: if the bowler doesn't bowl *very* well, the batsman will find it easier to score runs. When this happens, you'll see the fielders gradually being moved back, and a more defensive field-setting being adopted.

You'll probably have worked out for yourself that you're most likely to see an offensive (or attacking) field early in the game or early in a batsman's innings, because once he's settled he'll be seeing the ball more clearly and hitting it harder, so run-limitation becomes more important.

That's also why you rarely see an attacking field in the limited-over game (sometimes called the one-day game), because keeping down the number of runs scored by the opposition can be as important as getting them out.

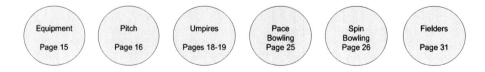

Equipment	Pitch	Umpires	Pace Bowling	Spin Bowling	Fielders
Page 15	Page 16	Pages 18-19	Page 25	Page 26	Page 31

Sometimes you'll see quite frenetic activity on the part of a fielder. The batsman hits the ball very hard, the fielder runs towards it, picks it up and throws it very fast towards the wicket-keeper, perhaps running the batsman out, perhaps not. Then, a moment later, you may see the same fielder strolling quite casually towards the ball and throwing it to the wicket-keeper in a gentle, looping curve, while the batsmen trot gently down the pitch to score a run.

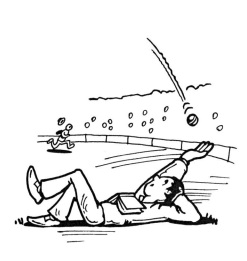

No point in wasting energy...

Why the difference in approach? Because the second time the ball was perhaps hit less hard, and the fielder realised he couldn't stop them scoring one run whatever he did. But he also knew that there was no chance of them even *trying* to score a second run, because he already had the ball in his hand; there was therefore no point in wasting energy he might very well need a few seconds later.

But there is another possible reason, a little more subtle. It may be that it was the last ball of an over, and the batsman who hit the ball has only just come in, whilst his partner has been in for a couple of hours and has already scored a lot of runs. If the new batsman is allowed to score a run off the last ball of an over, that means he'll go down to the other end, and therefore be receiving the bowling at the beginning of the next over – thus enabling the fielding side to keep the pressure on him.

There are in fact endless subtleties in the art of setting a field, but to go into them now would take us well out of the scope of this book. But let me give you one more typical example of what might happen.

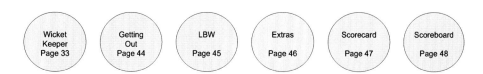

Wicket Keeper Page 33

Getting Out Page 44

LBW Page 45

Extras Page 46

Scorecard Page 47

Scoreboard Page 48

A bowler may know that a particular batsman likes to hit the ball on the *leg side*, especially if it's pitched short and reaches him at about shoulder height. When he does this, he usually keeps the ball down to avoid being caught, but sometimes, especially early in his innings, he may get his timing slightly wrong and hit the ball in the air. So a man will be placed on the *square-leg* boundary in case that happens. In the meantime, of course, the bowler will make sure that he occasionally gets the chance to play that shot.

The snag with that is that the batsman will know exactly what the bowler has in mind, because, of course, every time a fielder is moved, the batsman makes a mental note of where he's moved to. The only thing he doesn't know is when such a ball will come, and if, when it does come, it's coming very fast in the direction of his head, his attempts to take evasive action may very well have the result that the fielding side were looking for. Alternatively, he may accept the challenge and play the shot anyway; sometimes it works in the batsman's favour, sometimes it doesn't.

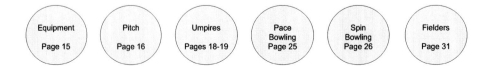

Equipment	Pitch	Umpires	Pace Bowling	Spin Bowling	Fielders
Page 15	Page 16	Pages 18-19	Page 25	Page 26	Page 31

Diversion 7 - Fielders

Something which newcomers to the game of cricket find strange is the names given to various fielding positions – names such as square leg, silly mid-on and gully, for instance. Like any activity – and not just sport – cricket has its own jargon, or shorthand, and it does not take long to understand, once you realise on what it is based.

We have already explained the terms leg side, on side and off side, so it doesn't take much imagination to work out on which side of the batsman a fielder called mid-off, or mid-on, or fine leg is standing. If someone refers to deep mid-off, then that indicates that he is standing well back (= deep), probably on the boundary. If he's called silly mid-off, he's standing close to the bat. With a cricket ball being as hard as it is, it's not difficult to see how that name came about! The origin of some names is lost in the mists of time. No one, for instance, is quite sure of the origins of the names point or gully, although everyone knows roughly where those players stand, and that is what really matters.

You will usually see some fielders (sometimes as many as four) standing behind the wicket, on the off-side, close to the wicket-keeper. These are known collectively as the slips, and they are frequently called upon to take very hard catches when the ball flies off the edge of the bat. Since this usually happens by accident, it's easy to see where this name comes from too.

You will find all the important names of fielding positions in the glossary, but on the next page you will find a diagram indicating where such fielders stand. The positions shown are by no means fixed, of course: the fielders may move about and cover quite a lot of ground. Bear in mind, though, that, leaving aside the bowler and wicket-keeper, you only have nine fielders to play with, so the placing of fielders can become a very difficult problem, and plays a big part in the bowling side's strategy.

In a limited-overs game you sometimes find restrictions on where fielders may be placed. You may see a ring marked on the field, for instance, and at certain times the fielding side may be obliged to have a certain number of fielders inside that ring. This is to prevent them from setting an extremely defensive field right from the start of the innings, and also to encourage the batting side to start scoring fast rather than waiting until they've settled in before trying to hit the ball hard, as they would in a first-class game.

Fielders Page 31
Fielders Page 31

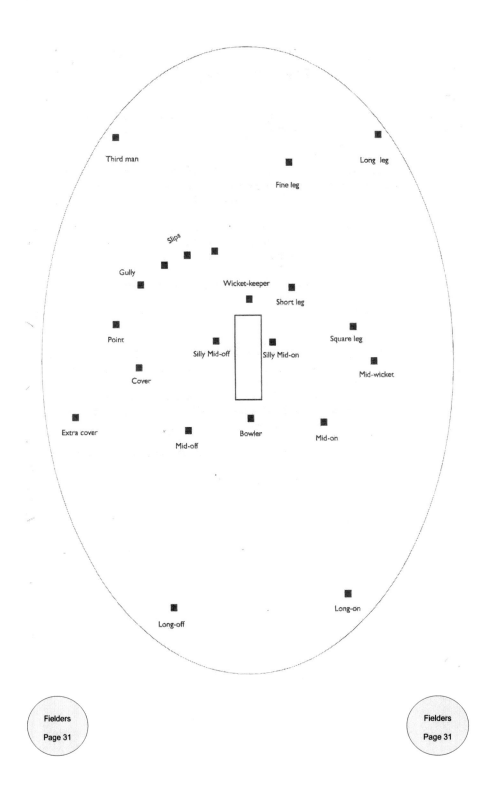

Diversion 8 - The Wicket-Keeper

A wicket-keeper needs good eyesight, great powers of concentration, and cat-like agility, for he is likely to be involved in the action virtually every time a ball is bowled, because even when the batsman hits the ball, the fielder who picks it up will invariably throw it back to the wicket-keeper.

Like the batsman, the wicket-keeper has to try and work out what the ball is going to do when it bounces. Unlike the batsman, however, he doesn't have the option of leaving it alone when it reaches him, because if he does, he's giving runs away to the other side.

He needs to be particularly alert when it comes to taking catches, because most catches that go to the wicket-keeper come off the edge of the bat, sometimes with only the faintest of contact being made, which can lead to controversy over whether the bat actually touched the ball or not.

When a fast bowler is in operation, the wicket-keeper usually stands well back from the stumps, but for a slow (or sometimes even for a medium-pace) bowler, he will stand up close, because there is a chance then of the batsman being deceived by the flight of the ball or by the spin, and being out of his ground when the ball reaches the wicket-keeper, in which case he breaks the wicket with the ball (or even with his hand or arm, provided he is actually holding the ball at the time), and the batsman is then out stumped.

A good wicket-keeper will also keep talking to the bowler and his captain, because he is in the best position to see the ball from the batsman's point of view, and so he is able to make suggestions about where to bowl, where to place fielders, etc.

Wicket Keeper Page 33

Wicket Keeper Page 33

Chapter 5 – More about batting

What has been said about bowling and fielding will already have given you some idea of the problems faced by the batsman, but there are others besides, not least those caused by the batsman's own state of mind, because one of the key ingredients in building a successful innings is concentration. There are few games where one lapse of concentration, one unforced error, can not only cause great problems for yourself and for your team, but can rule you out of the game altogether.

The batsman's objective is, basically, to score as many runs as possible. In order to achieve that, he must obviously make sure the bowler doesn't get him out before he's accumulated those runs. That means that, at least some of the time, the batsman isn't trying to score runs at all – he's just trying to avoid getting out. In other words, like the bowler and the fielders, the batsman will be operating sometimes in *defensive* mode, sometimes in *attacking* mode, and this will depend largely on the way the bowler bowls.

In most games the best players calculate the risks that are worth taking. A top tennis player will decline to play the shot which seems most obvious to the ordinary club player, because he realises that it will only work perhaps two or three times out of ten, whereas another shot may be safer. Similarly a golfer may decide against driving over water or between trees, because he calculates that the odds would be against the shot being successful.

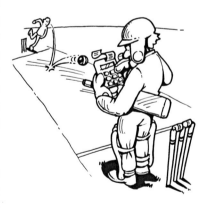

And so it is with batting. Each time the ball is bowled, the batsman has to decide which shot is safest. 'I might hit this for four,' he will think, 'but if I just clip it with the edge instead of middling it, there are four men standing there waiting for a catch, and if I'm out now, the team will be in a real mess.'

The best players
calculate the risks

As I made clear above, the batsman takes care to memorise where the fielders are stationed; if, therefore, he's aware that there is no one standing in the right position to take such a catch, he is more likely to go ahead with the shot.

So the first thing a batsman must do is decide whether he needs to play a defensive or an attacking shot. But, as in most games involving a moving ball, it's no good deciding beforehand which shot you're going to play; if you do, you may occasionally get lucky and get away with it, but most of the time your chances of having selected the right shot in advance are little better than those of winning the National Lottery jackpot.

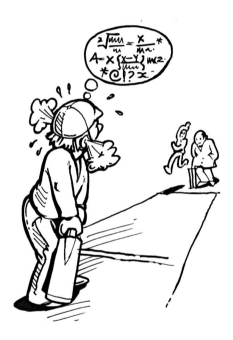

You have less than a second...

What that means in effect is that you have less than a second – maybe as little as half a second – to try to assess the *line* and *length*, *speed* and *bounce* of the delivery before you decide what shot to play.

Misjudge any of these factors, and you could easily be out. The good batsman, of course, will know roughly what sort of delivery to expect from any given bowler, but, as we have seen, that bowler is able to introduce a number of variables, and that means the batsman needs to assess from the way the bowler runs up, the way his arm comes over and – if the bowler doesn't conceal it too effectively – the way he's gripping the ball, what kind of delivery is on its way.

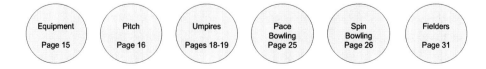

Equipment	Pitch	Umpires	Pace Bowling	Spin Bowling	Fielders
Page 15	Page 16	Pages 18-19	Page 25	Page 26	Page 31

In the meantime, as I have already said, he will also have made a mental note of where the fielders are placed, because he needs first of all to avoid playing the ball in such a way that one of them can catch it. Secondly, if he wants to score runs, he needs to hit the ball into whatever gap he can find. You'll often find, in fact, that if the batsman hits the ball very hard, but straight to a fielder, he doesn't score anything at all, but if he hits it gently into a gap between two fielders, he may very well score two.

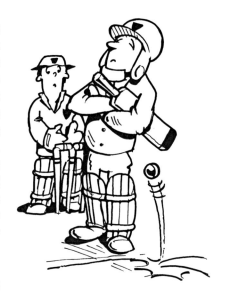

Sometimes you'll even see a batsman playing no shot at all, especially when facing a fast bowler. If the ball is coming fast, bounces some way down the pitch, and is still rising when it reaches the batsman, it's wiser not to try to hit it at all, because the odds

The batsman constantly refuses to play a shot...

are against you. The exception to this, of course, would be if the ball is going to hit your stumps if you don't put your bat in the way!

This is one of the things that can make the game boring. If a fast bowler is constantly hurling the ball very fast but outside the line of the off stump, and the batsman equally constantly refuses to play a shot, then nothing happens, and both game and spectators go to sleep.

This, incidentally, is almost always the bowler's fault, because he has stopped forcing the batsman to make decisions. What is really important is for the bowler to create doubt in the batsman's mind, either in terms of length or direction. The batsman must be made to wonder whether it's safe for him not to play a shot, or he must be made to hesitate between moving forward to play the ball or moving back.

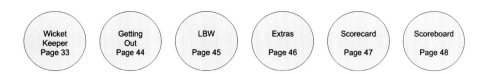

Wicket Keeper Page 33 | Getting Out Page 44 | LBW Page 45 | Extras Page 46 | Scorecard Page 47 | Scoreboard Page 48

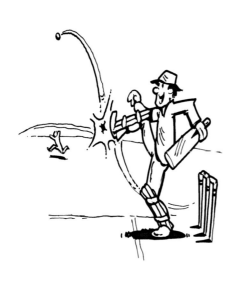

Playing off the front foot...

It's the creation of such uncertainty which characterizes a good bowling performance. So, when you hear a commentator talking about a batsman being 'in two minds', it either means that the batsman is unusually incompetent or that the bowler is bowling well.

There are lots of different shots a batsman can play. We've already seen that there is a choice between playing 'off the front foot' and playing 'off the back foot'. As far as defence is concerned, that's just about all there is to it. If you play these defensive shots perfectly every time, then, at least in theory, you'll never get out. On the other hand, you'll never score any runs either, so your contribution to your team's effort might still not be very significant.

As far as the recognised attacking shots are concerned, these all have special names, derived either from the area of the field into which they're hit or from the nature of the shot itself – or sometimes both. You'll find definitions of these in the *Glossary*, so I won't take up space by defining them all now. Here is a list of the major ones:

Cut: *Late cut, Square cut*

Drive: *Cover-drive, Off-drive, On-drive, Square drive, Straight drive*

Hook, Pull, Sweep: These are all methods of hitting a short ball to the leg side. There are differences between these shots, but they are all very similar, and we don't need to differentiate between them here, except to say that a *reverse sweep* is one where a right-handed batsman plays the shot as if he were a left-hander, or vice-versa.

Leg Glance

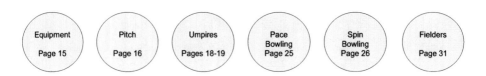

Equipment Page 15 | Pitch Page 16 | Umpires Pages 18-19 | Pace Bowling Page 25 | Spin Bowling Page 26 | Fielders Page 31

These, of course, are deliberate, recognised shots. Sometimes a batsman touches the ball and it flies off the edge of the bat and goes in a direction he never intended. This is sometimes called a '*snick*' or an '*edge*', and of course it's risky because the batsman is not in control of the shot and he may very well be out caught.

Sometimes a (not very good) batsman will just swing the bat blindly and hope for the best. He may be lucky and hit the ball for four or six, but more often than not he'll be out. For some reason this type of play is sometimes called 'agricultural', or 'a cow-shot' – probably because it's the sort of shot you're more likely to find in a match being played between yokels on a village green than in a test match at Lord's, although, even in serious cricket, there's an area of the field which many people call 'cow corner', because it's the area where cow shots are most likely to end up. (If you look at the diagram in the Diversion on Fielding, it's on the boundary somewhere between Mid-on and Long-on.)

The batsman is allowed to use his legs, but there is always a risk involved in doing that (see the Diversion on Leg Before Wicket), and he is not allowed to score runs if he plays the ball deliberately with his leg or foot.

Another important feature of batting is the matter of *calling*. As you know, a run is only scored when both batsmen have run to the other end of the pitch. This means that each batsman has to know what the other man's intentions are, so a system of 'calling' is used. Generally speaking, if the batsman hits the ball in front of the wicket, he's in a better position to judge whether it's safe to run or not, so it's his responsibility to 'call'. If the ball goes behind the wicket, the non-striker is in a better position to judge, so it's regarded as being his 'call'. But disagreements sometimes occur.

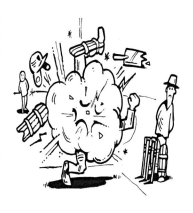

Disagreements sometimes occur...

| Wicket Keeper Page 33 | Getting Out Page 44 | LBW Page 45 | Extras Page 46 | Scorecard Page 47 | Scoreboard Page 48 |

Usually, you'll hear one or other of the batsmen shout 'Yes!', 'No!' or 'Wait!' – or something along those lines. If his partner is not listening, or if he thinks the other batsman's call is too risky, things can go badly wrong; you can have situations where both batsmen find themselves at the same end, with the result that one of them will be given out – assuming, that is, that a fielder has gathered the ball and 'broken' his wicket before he can retrieve his proper position. This tends to be followed by another traditional call: 'Sorry!'

I don't need in a book like this to go into great detail where the tactics of batting are concerned, but it will have become clear to you by now that there are some occasions when scoring runs is important, and others where it is really more important to make sure that you don't get out.

In a limited-overs match you don't normally have time for such niceties though. You've only got a certain number of balls to face, and you know pretty well how many runs you need to score – in fact, in the case of the side batting second, you know exactly how many runs you need to score. (There's one exception to this, which I shall deal with in a moment.)

But not only do you know how many runs you need to score, you also know that if you don't score them, you're going to lose, whether you're out or not. So you have in mind roughly how many runs you need to score off every over, and you try to keep up with that pace (known as the *required run rate*) as best you can.

A similar situation can occur in the first-class game (when each side has two innings), when the batting side know how many runs they need to win, and how much time remains. But they might also know that they have two hours left to play, they need 300 runs to win, and have only three wickets left to fall, and that is a virtually impossible position from which to win. Since, in this form of cricket, a draw is declared if neither side actually wins, and it's considered better to draw than to lose, such a side would invariably try to hold out for a draw. That being so, the tactic would be just to concentrate on not getting out, because the number of runs scored would then be irrelevant.

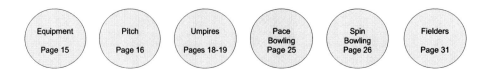

| Equipment | Pitch | Umpires | Pace Bowling | Spin Bowling | Fielders |
| Page 15 | Page 16 | Pages 18-19 | Page 25 | Page 26 | Page 31 |

This wouldn't necessarily lead to boring play though, because the fielding side, realising that giving away runs was now irrelevant, would set a very attacking field with a view to taking those final wickets, which would allow them to win the game, and the last hour or two of the game could become very exciting indeed.

In such a situation you might find one very good batsman batting alongside one who is not very good at all, and the good batsman will therefore try to make sure that he monopolises the bowling. (This is also known as 'farming' the bowling.) He will do that by trying to score a single off the fifth or sixth ball of every over so that he will be 'on strike' at the beginning of the next over.

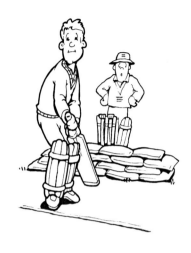

Just concentrate on not getting out...

Naturally, the fielding side will react to this by giving him the opportunity to score a run early in the over, which would mean that they will be able to bowl at the more vulnerable batsman. But the batsmen are not obliged to run if they don't want to.

It can also happen that one of the two batsmen can play spin bowling more easily than his colleague. In that case, if a spin bowler was operating from one end and a fast bowler from the other, the batsmen might try to organise their scoring so that each of them spent as much time as possible facing the type of bowling with which he felt most comfortable.

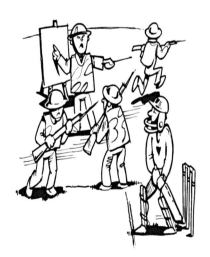

Setting an attacking field...

Wicket Keeper Page 33

Getting Out Page 44

LBW Page 45

Extras Page 46

Scorecard Page 47

Scoreboard Page 48

In other words, if you see batsmen not running when runs are apparently there for the taking, there is usually a good reason for it, and part of the enjoyment of watching cricket is to try and follow the psychological battle that lies behind the action you actually see on the field. One might even say that that is the main enjoyment, because to someone who does not appreciate that aspect of it, cricket really can be a boring game.

The implication is that cricket is an aggressive game, and so it is, but that aggression is usually channelled into playing according to the rules, not into breaking them, as one finds in some other games, and in cricket more than any other sport, the matter of 'playing the game' is synonymous with playing fairly.

(Somewhat paradoxically however, the concept of a 'level playing field' seems not to apply in cricket: if you go to watch a match at Lord's, for many years the indisputable headquarters of world cricket, it will at once become apparent to you that the playing surface has a significant slope – one side is nine feet higher than the other!)

Now for the exception I referred to above. As I said earlier, there is always a winner and a loser in a limited-overs match, but what happens if the match is obliged to end before a result can be declared? After all, it is just as likely to rain on a one-day limited-overs match as on an individual day of a test match.

If it rains so hard all day that no play is possible whatever, then no system could be conceived which would produce a worthy winner. But very often a match is simply shortened because of rain.

Let me give you an example: England are playing against Australia, and bat first. They score 272 in their allotted fifty overs, and then it's starts to rain. Three hours later conditions become playable once more, but so much time has been lost that there is only time for Australia to bat for twenty-five overs, not fifty. It is clearly unfair to expect Australia to score 273 to win in 25 overs.

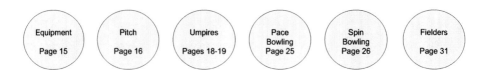

Equipment	Pitch	Umpires	Pace Bowling	Spin Bowling	Fielders
Page 15	Page 16	Pages 18-19	Page 25	Page 26	Page 31

In 1995 or thereabouts, two British statisticians, Frank Duckworth and Tony Lewis, devised a method of recalculating the target in such a case, a method which they claimed was fair, because it takes into account such things as the fact that a high run-rate is easier to maintain for, say, 20 overs than for 50, that lower-order batsmen can achieve less than those who go in first, etc.

The result of their work was that their system was introduced all over the world, and is now used in all international matches where a fair result would otherwise be impossible to achieve. Of course there are some people who complain about individual applications of the method, but it is generally accepted as being fair, and, in tribute to the system's creators, it is now known simply as Duckworth-Lewis, or the D/L method. It is incredibly complicated - the majority of players and spectators have no idea whatever of how it works - and, fortunately for me, I don't really need to explain it in a book like this!

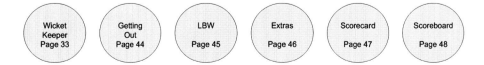

Wicket Keeper Page 33

Getting Out Page 44

LBW Page 45

Extras Page 46

Scorecard Page 47

Scoreboard Page 48

Diversion 9 - Ways of getting out

There are a number of ways in which a batsman may be dismissed, some of them much more common than others.

Bowled: When the ball hits the wicket and dislodges at least one of the bails, whether or not the batsman has first touched it with his bat or part of his body.

Caught: When the ball touches the batsman's bat or hand, and is then caught by a fielder before it touches the ground.

Leg before wicket (LBW): When the ball would have hit the stumps if the batsman's leg or another part of his body hadn't prevented it, the batsman may be out. But this is very complicated, and is dealt with in detail on the next page.

Stumped: If the batsman, in receiving the ball, is out of his ground and the wicket-keeper breaks the wicket with the ball, then he is out stumped – unless he is out of his ground because he is trying to score a run, in which case he is run out.

Hit wicket: If, while in the act of playing, or just after playing a shot, the batsman breaks his own wicket with the bat, part of his body or part of his equipment, then he is out hit wicket.

In the case of all these dismissals, the bowler gets the credit. There are, however, five other ways of being out, for which the bowler does not get the credit. The first four are extremely rare:

Handled the ball: This does not mean the batsman can't pick the ball up to pass it to a fielder once it has gone 'dead', i.e. when all activity consequent on the bowling of a delivery has finished and all that needs to be done is for the ball to be passed back to the bowler for him to start again. It simply means that he cannot deliberately play the ball with his hand to stop himself being out in any other way.

Obstructing the field: Preventing a fielder from catching, stopping or picking up the ball.

Hit the ball twice: The batsman is allowed to hit the ball a second time to stop it going on to his stumps, but not to prevent someone catching it or to score a run.

Timed out: When an incoming batsman deliberately delays the resumption of play.

Much more common, especially in limited-over games when the batsmen take risks when trying to score runs quickly is:

Getting Out Page 44

Run out: When either batsman is attempting a run and the fielding side break the wicket with the ball while he is still out of his ground.

Getting Out Page 44

Diversion 10 - Leg before wicket (L.B.W.)

This is one of the most frequent ways in which a batsman may be out, and one of the most difficult to understand. It is easy enough to understand how it was first decided that playing the ball with your legs to stop it hitting the wicket was illegal, but not so easy to see the reasoning behind the law which has gradually evolved to cope with many generations of batsmen trying to bend the law as much as possible.

It is also a dismissal constantly surrounded by controversy, because whether the decision is justified or not is entirely a matter for the judgment of the umpire who stands at the bowler's end, since nobody else on the field, and certainly not the batsman, the bowler, or even the wicket keeper, is in a position to assess the different criteria which have to be considered.

These are the questions which an umpire must ask himself:

(i) Would the ball have gone on to hit the wicket if the batsman's leg (or any part of the body) had not been in the way? If the answer is 'no', then he must give the batsman 'not out'. If the answer is 'yes', he considers the second question.

(ii) Did the ball pitch outside the batsman's leg stump? If the answer is 'yes', he must give the batsman 'not out'. If it is 'no', he considers the third question.

(iii) Did the ball pitch in line with the stumps? If the answer is 'yes', then he must give the batsman 'out'. If the answer is 'no', he considers the fourth question.

(iv) The ball then must have pitched outside the batsman's off stump. Did he make any attempt to hit the ball? If the answer to that is 'yes', then he must give the batsman 'not out'. If the answer is 'no', he must give him out.

As you can see this is all extremely complicated. In fact there is a further complication: in deciding whether the ball would have hit the stumps or not, the umpire must take into account whether the ball was swinging or spinning, and what the effect of that would have been. Fortunately for the umpire, he is protected by the laws which add to all these questions the crucial words 'in the opinion of the umpire'! Even so, this decision may be, and often is, subject to review under the DRS system.

The umpire will only adjudicate if the fielding side appeals by shouting 'How's that?'. If he seems to take a long time to give his decision, that's because he has to ask himself all those questions before he can say 'out' or 'not out'.

LBW
Page 45

LBW
Page 45

Diversion 11 - Extras

Sometimes runs are added to the batting side's score but are not credited to the batsman because he didn't hit the ball with his bat; these runs are called extras. There are four kinds of extras:

Wide: when the bowler bowls the ball so wide (or so high) that the batsman can't reach it, the umpire calls 'wide', and signals this decision by holding out both arms horizontally. One run is added to the score, unless the batsmen run or the ball crosses the boundary, in which case all the runs scored are classed as extras. In limited-over matches the umpires are much stricter over their interpretation of what constitutes a wide.

No-ball: If the umpire is not satisfied that part of the bowler's front foot was behind the popping crease when he bowled (i.e. in the batsman's 'ground'), or he thinks the bowler's back foot touched or was outside the return crease, he calls 'no-ball' and one run is added to the score. He also signals 'no-ball' by holding out one arm horizontally. A no-ball may also be called if either umpire thinks the bowler is throwing rather than bowling the ball. If the batsman hits a no-ball and scores runs from it, those runs are credited to the batsman.

In the case of both wides and no-balls an extra ball is added to the over. With the exception of being run out while attempting a run, and some other instances which are so rare they needn't concern us here, a batsman can't be out off a no-ball or a wide.

Bye: If the ball passes both the bat and the wicket (without the batsman touching it), and the wicket-keeper fails to stop it, runs may be scored in the normal way. These count as 'byes', and the umpire signals them by raising his open hand above his head.

Leg-bye: This is exactly the same as a bye except that the ball will have touched part of the batsman's body as he tried to hit it. A leg-bye, which is not allowed if the umpire thinks the batsman wasn't really trying to hit the ball with his bat, is signalled by tapping his leg.

There is one other rather unusual circumstance in which extra runs may be scored. Sometimes a close fielder will wear a protective helmet, and when this is no longer needed, it will be placed on the ground somewhere out of the way (usually behind the wicket-keeper). If the ball should then strike the helmet, five runs are added to the batting side's score, either as extras or as runs credited to the batsman if the batsman actually hit the ball.

Extras
Page 46

Extras
Page 46

Diversion 12 - Scorecard

The scorecard gives you all the details you need to know about a match. It lists all the players in each team, showing in what order they batted, how they were out, and how many runs they scored. It also shows the total score, what the score was when each batsman was out, and gives details of each bowler's performance. And of course it tells you the result. Here is a scorecard for a 50-over match between England and Australia:

AUSTRALIA			ENGLAND		
* M.A.Taylor	b Cork	2	* M.A.Atherton	lbw b McDermott	1
M.E.Waugh	lbw b Gough	13	† A.J.Stewart	not out	104
R.T. Ponting	c Stewart b Cork	22	N.Hussein	run out	43
S.R.Waugh	st Stewart b Croft	65	G.P.Thorpe	not out	36
S.G.Law	c Thorpe b Caddick	7	G.A.Hick		
M.G.Bevan	c Hussein b Gough	14	A.J.Hollioake		
S.Lee	b Tufnell	18	D.G.Cork		
† I.A. Healey	lbw b Croft	27	D.Gough		
S.K.Warne	b Tufnell	0	R.D.B.Croft		
C.J.McDermott	not out	7	A.R.Caddick		
G.D.McGrath	not out	5	P.C.R.Tufnell		
Extras	b2, l-b3, w1, n-b3	9	Extras	b4, n-b2	6
Total	(9 wkts, 50 overs)	189	Total	(2 wkts, 41.2 overs)	190

Fall of wickets: 1-2, 2-31, 3-66, 4-82, 5-104, 6-134, 7-159, 8-159, 9-177

Fall of wickets: 1-2, 2-97

England bowling: Cork 10-1-45-2 (In-b), Gough 10-1-37-2 (1n-b,1w), Caddick 10-1-32-1, Croft 10-2-31-2, Tufnell 10-1-39-2 (1 n-b).

Australia bowling: McDermott 7-1-35-1 (1 n-b), McGrath 7-0-41-0 (1 n-b), Warne 10-1-49-0, Lee 4.2-0-19-0, M.E.Waugh 7-1-18-0, S.R.Waugh 6-0-24-0.

ENGLAND WON BY EIGHT WICKETS

* indicates the captain of the team; † indicates the wicket-keeper.

Australia scored 189 in their allotted 50 overs, losing 9 wickets in the process. England passed the Australian score in 41.2 overs (41 overs and 2 balls), and only lost 2 wickets. So England won by 8 wickets, having 8 wickets still to fall when they passed the Australian score, and the last seven batsmen were not needed. The first Australian wicket fell with the score at only 2, the second when they had scored 31, the third at 66, etc.

In the Australian innings, Ponting was caught by wicket-keeper Stewart off the bowling of Cork; S.R. Waugh was stumped by Stewart off the bowling of Croft; the other dismissals are self-explanatory.

Bowling: Take Gough as an example: he bowled 10 overs, including 1 maiden, conceded 37 runs, took 2 wickets, bowled 1 no-ball and 1 wide.

48

Diversion 13 - Scoreboard

On every cricket ground you will see a scoreboard, which enables the spectators and players to see the current score. Sometimes the scorer can be seen sitting at a window in the middle of the scoreboard. This illustration shows the scoreboard as it would have been shortly after the fall of England's first wicket in the match detailed on page 47.

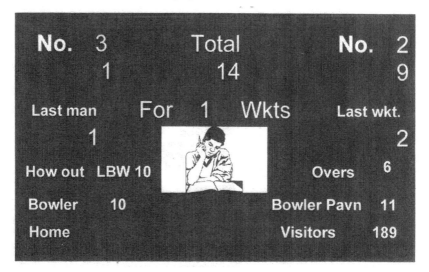

It shows that so far 14 runs have been scored, and one wicket has fallen. The current batsmen, no. 3 (Hussein) and no. 2 (Stewart), have so far scored 1 and 9 respectively. The last man out scored 1, and the score when he was out was 2. Beneath his score you will see that he was out lbw to the bowling of no. 10, McDermott. In the Australian innings, S.R. Waugh would have been shown st2b9, i.e. stumped by Stewart off the bowling of Croft, whilst Law would have been shown c4b10 (caught by Thorpe off the bowling of Caddick).

On the right you will see that the England innings has now been in progress for 6 overs. Below that you will see that the current bowlers are no. 10 (McDermott) and (at the Pavilion end) no. 11 (McGrath). Finally there is a reminder that Australia scored 189 in their innings.

At some of the biggest grounds the scoreboard is more elaborate, but also simpler to interpret because the players are identified by name. Such scoreboards may also identify who has just fielded the ball, and give details of each bowler's performance.

Scoreboard Page 48

Scoreboard Page 48

6 - Glossary

All-rounder A player who is good at both batting and bowling.

Appeal A request by the fielding side to the umpire to declare a batsman out. Usually takes the form of a shout 'How's that?'.

Ashes A mythical trophy which goes to the winners of a series of matches between England and Australia.

Asking rate The number of runs per over a batting side needs to score on average if they are to win the game.

Bail One of two small pieces of wood which are placed on top of the three stumps which form the wicket, and which must be removed if the wicket is to be judged broken.

Bat-pad If the ball hits the batsman's pad, and then his bat (or vice versa), and the ball is then caught by a fielder, this is known as a bat-pad catch. A fielder standing in a position which would allow him to take such a catch is said to be in bat-pad position.

Batting average An indication of a batsman's performance over, say, a season — or over his entire career — which consists of dividing the total number of runs he has scored by the number of times he has been out, thus giving the average score he makes in each innings.

Beamer A full toss which is aimed straight at the head of a batsman. This really only happens by accident, because such a ball would be declared by the umpire to be a no-ball, and the bowler warned.

Block-hole The point on the pitch where the batsman rests the tip of his bat while waiting for the ball to be delivered.

Bouncer A fast, short-pitched ball, which bounces at least chest-high.

Boundary (i) A line marking the limits of the field of play.

Boundary(ii) A ball which passes over this boundary either without bouncing, thus scoring six, or having bounced at least once, thus scoring four. A boundary is signalled by the umpire raising both hands above his head for a six or waving one arm from side to side for a four.

Bowling analysis An indication of a bowler's performance in a given innings, which shows the number of overs he has bowled, how many of those overs were maidens, how many runs were scored off him, and how many wickets he took.

Bump ball A ball which looks as if it has gone straight off the bat to a fielder without bouncing, but which was actually played straight down onto the ground, and then ballooned into the air. (Sometimes called a 'Crowd Catch')

Bye A run taken by the batsmen when the ball has gone past the wicket-keeper without touching the bat. The umpire signals a bye by raising one hand above his head.

Call An indication by one batsman that he wants the other batsman to run. The normal convention is that, if the ball is hit in front of the striker it is the striker's decision whether to run (and therefore he should call), but if it goes behind him, the call to run should be given by the non-striker.

Century A score of one hundred runs or more made by a single batsman in a single innings.

Cover A fielding position, in which the fielder stands roughly half way between the batsman and the boundary, on the off side, at an angle of approximately 45°. Also known as cover point.

Crease A white line marked on the pitch. There are four creases at each end: the bowling crease, which is the line on which the wicket itself is placed, the two return creases, one on either side of the wicket, which indicate the area from which the bowler is allowed to deliver the ball, and the popping crease, which is the line in front of the wicket on which the batsman normally stands to receive the ball.

Cut A way of hitting the ball, on the off side, which will send it either square of the wicket (a square cut) or behind the wicket (a late cut).

Cutter A leg-cutter and an off-cutter are similar to leg-breaks and off-breaks, but bowled much faster.

Declaration The captain of a batting side may declare his side's innings closed at any time he wishes. The act of doing this is called a declaration.

Deep A fielder standing a long way from the bat, e.g. on the boundary, is said to be fielding in the deep.

Dot ball A ball from which no run is scored, so-called because the scorer records this by putting a dot in the score-book.

Drive A hard-hit shot in front of the wicket. Depending on the direction in which the ball travels, it may be called an on-drive, an off-drive, a cover drive, or even a square drive.

Duck When a batsman is out without scoring, he is said to have made a duck. When he scores his first run he is said to have broken his duck.

Edge If the batsman does not hit the ball cleanly it can fly off the edge of the bat, and this will frequently result in a catch either by the wicket-keeper, the slips, or short leg. Sometimes there may be the finest of touches: this is called a thin edge; if more positive contact is made, it is called a thick edge. The inside edge is the one nearer the batsman, the outside edge the edge further away.

Extra cover A fielding position similar to that of cover, but deeper.

Extras Runs which are added to a side's score, but are not credited to an individual batsman, e.g. byes, leg byes, no-balls and wides.

Fine leg A fielder standing on the leg side, behind the wicket, about half way between the wicket and the boundary.

Follow-on In a two-innings match, the side batting second may be asked to bat again (follow on) if their score is a long way short of the other side's first innings total (150 or 200 runs, depending on the type of match).

Follow-through The continuation of a bowler's action after delivery.

Foot marks Marks made on the pitch by the bowlers as they follow through. These can cause great problems for the batsman, because a ball pitching in a foot mark can behave in a quite unpredictable fashion.

Full toss A ball which reaches the batsman without bouncing.

Googly A ball which looks as if it is going to turn from leg to off, but in fact does the opposite, thus deceiving the batsman.

Guard When a batsman begins his innings he takes guard by making a mark on the pitch in order to make sure he is standing in the right place to receive the ball. Before making this mark, he will ask the umpire to help him.

Gully A fielding position on the off side, fairly close to the bat and roughly equivalent to fourth or fifth slip.

Half-volley A ball which bounces just in front of the bat, and is therefore fairly easy to hit hard.

Hat trick The taking of three wickets by the same bowler in the space of three balls (not necessarily in the same over).

Hit wicket If a batsman hits or treads on his own wicket while playing a shot, he is adjudged to be out Hit wicket.

Hook Shot played by a batsman to a short-pitched ball on the leg side, whereby he hooks it in the direction of the leg-side boundary.

Innings (i) the time during which a batsman is in.

Innings (ii) the time during which a side is in.

Interval A break in play. Traditionally there are two breaks in play, the lunch interval and the tea interval, although there may be different arrangements for a limited-overs match. There is also a ten-minute interval between the end of one side's innings and the beginning of the next.

LBW See Leg before wicket

Leg before wicket A batsman may be given out leg before wicket (LBW) if, whether by accident or design, he prevents the ball from hitting his wicket by playing it with any part of his body. The conditions for this are somewhat complicated, however, and are discussed in the Diversion entitled LBW.

Leg break A ball which, after pitching, turns from the leg-side towards the offside.

Leg bye A run taken by the batsmen when the ball has not touched the bat but has come into contact with part of the batsman's body (not necessarily the leg). A leg-bye is only allowed if the umpire considers the batsman was genuinely trying to hit the ball. The umpire signals a leg-bye by tapping his leg.

Leg glance A shot played by the batsman to a ball about to hit his legs, where he turns his bat so that the ball is deflected behind him, on the leg side.

Leg side The side on which the batsman's legs are positioned as he stands to receive the ball.

Length An indication of the point where a bowler pitches the ball when bowling.

Limited-over A limited-over match is one where the amount of time available to each side for batting is set beforehand, each side, for instance, having fifty overs in which to bat.

Line The direction in which a bowler bowls.

Long hop A ball pitched so short that it is easy for the batsman to hit.

Long-leg A fielding position, similar to Fine leg, but on the boundary.

Long-off A fielding position, similar to Mid-off, but on the boundary.

Long-on A fielding position, similar to Mid-on, but on the boundary.

Maiden An over during the course of which no runs are scored.

Mark, off the A batsman is said to be off the mark when he scores his first run.

Mid-on A fielding position in front of the batsman, on the leg (or on) side, about thirty yards or so from the bat.

Mid-off A fielding position in front of the batsman, on the off side, about thirty yards or so from the bat.

Mid-wicket A fielder occupying a similar position to that of cover point, but on the leg side.

Nets A practice area, surrounded by nets so that the ball does not travel a long way when hit, thus eliminating the need for fielders. When a batsman speaks of having a net he means having a practice session in the nets.

New ball In all first-class matches the bowling side is allowed to use a new ball after a certain number of overs have been bowled with the old one. This is a distinct advantage, because a new ball is shinier, and therefore more likely to swing in the air.

Night-watchman If a wicket falls shortly before the close of play a captain sometimes chooses not to send one of his best batsman in to bat, but sends someone in instead whose job is just to stay there and make sure no further wicket falls before the close of play. This player is called a night-watchman.

No-ball If a bowler oversteps the popping crease, the umpire calls No-ball, one ball is added to the over, and one run is added to the score. If the batsman hits a no-ball, however, any runs scored are credited to the batsman. The only way in which a batsman may be given out off a no-ball is Run out. The umpire signals a no-ball by raising his left arm horizontally.

Off-break A ball which, after pitching, turns from the off side towards the leg side.

Off side Opposite to the leg side or on side.

On side Another term for the leg side; the side on which the batsman's legs are positioned as he stands to receive the ball. This will vary according to whether the batsman is right-handed or left-handed.

Over A series of six deliveries, each bowled by the same bowler.

Overthrow If a fielder throws the ball back towards the stumps and it is not stopped by the wicket keeper, the bowler, or by another fielder, the batsmen may continue to run, and these runs are called overthrows.

Pair A batsman scores a pair when he fails to score in either innings of a match. He is said to be on a pair at the start of his second innings if he failed to score in the first. A king pair involves being out first ball in both innings of a match.

Pitch The bowling and batting area of the field, 22 yards long.

Point A fielder close to the bat on the off-side, standing roughly square to the batsman.

Popping crease See crease.

Pull A shot played by a batsman to a ball pitched on the off side, which he pulls in the direction of the leg-side boundary.

Retired hurt A batsman who is injured may be replaced by another batsman. If later on (but only at the fall of a wicket) he is able to resume, he may do so. If he is not able to resume he is designated retired hurt in the score-book, and is considered not out.

Run out If, when attempting a run, a batsman fails to cross the popping crease before the ball, having been thrown by a fielder, hits the wicket, he is given out Run out. Such a dismissal is not credited to the bowler.

Scorer The person who writes down the score, recording the result of every ball bowled.

Scoring rate An indication of the progress of the batting side, achieved by dividing the number of runs scored by the number of overs bowled so far. The scoring rate is also sometimes expressed in the number of runs scored per 100 balls bowled.

Seam (i) The stitching which joins together the two halves of a cricket ball.

Seam (ii) A type of bowling in which the bowler uses the seam of the ball to make the ball change direction, either in flight or on landing.

Short leg A close fielder on the leg side.

Sight-screen A white screen or board placed at either end of the ground which provides a contrasting background, making it easier for the batsman to see the ball.(Or a black screen when a white ball is used, as happens in professional one-day games.)

Signal The way in which umpires convey their decisions to the scorer.

Silly Used in conjunction with the name of a fielding position to indicate that the fielder is standing closer to the bat than would normally be the case, e.g. silly point, silly mid-on, etc.

Single When a batsman hits the ball and one run is scored, that run is referred to as a single.

Slips Close fielders standing on the off side, behind the bat, positioned to catch balls which the wicket-keeper cannot reach. Occasionally you will hear a reference to a leg slip, when a fielder is placed in a similar position to slip but on the leg side. It is not easy, however, to say exactly how a leg slip differs from a fine leg.

Spell A series of overs bowled by one bowler: if a bowler bowls eight consecutive overs before giving way to someone else, he is said to have had an eight-over spell.

Splice A cricket bat is made up of two parts, the handle and the blade. The splice is the v-shaped section where the handle and the blade are joined.

Square leg A fielder standing on the leg side, square of the batsman.

Sticky wicket Very rarely found these days in the first-class game because pitches are covered as soon as rain starts to fall. In the days when pitches were left uncovered, the effect of sunshine on a wet pitch was to make it easier for spin-bowlers to turn the ball, making life extremely difficult even for the very best batsmen. A pitch in this condition was called a sticky wicket.

Strike rate A measure of a bowler's performance, either in an individual innings or match, or a season, or an entire career. It is calculated by multiplying the number of overs he has bowled by six (i.e. to show the number of balls bowled) and dividing that number by the number of wickets he has taken. Thus a bowler with a strike rate of 37.2 has, on average, taken one wicket in every 37.2 balls bowled.

Stump One of three sticks placed upright at either end of the pitch to form the wicket.

Stumped If a batsman fails to hit the ball, and the wicket-keeper is able to break the wicket with the ball while the batsman is out of his ground (i.e. with no part of him or his bat touching the ground behind the popping crease) the umpire may give him out stumped.

Sweep A shot somewhat similar to a pull, but involving a sweeping action.

Tail-ender One of the last batsmen in a team to bat, and hence one who is probably not a very effective batsman.

Test match A match between two of the major cricket-playing countries.

Third man A fielder standing roughly in the same position as the slips in relation to the batsman, but much nearer the boundary.

Toss Before a match begins the two captains toss a coin to decide which side will bat first. Since the weather and the condition of the pitch play an important part in the game, winning the toss can be crucial.

Twelfth man A reserve player, who is not allowed to bat or bowl, but who can take the place of an injured fielder.

Umpire There are two umpires who control the game, one standing at the bowler's end, just behind the wicket, the other standing at square leg.

Uneven bounce On a good pitch the batsman should be able to assume that the ball will bounce predictably. Sometimes, however, two balls may be bowled which look as if they should behave identically, but one bounces and the other doesn't, which makes batting (and wicket-keeping) very difficult. Also called variable bounce.

Wicket (i) The three stumps, surmounted by bails, which the bowler has to try and hit and the batsman has to defend.

Wicket (ii) Another term for the pitch itself.

Wicket (iii) The dismissal of a batsman.

Wicket-keeper A fielder who stands behind the wicket and whose main job is to catch the ball if the batsman does not touch it.

Wide A ball which is bowled so wide that the batsman cannot reach it. This adds one run to the score, and an extra ball is added to the over. The umpire signals the calling of a wide by stretching both arms out wide. The umpires are much stricter over the bowling of wides in limited-over matches.

Yorker A ball which pitches in the batsman's block-hole and which, if the batsman doesn't take extreme care, may go under his bat and hit his stumps.

7 – Conclusion

If you've got as far as this, you now know enough about cricket to have some idea of what's going on if you watch a game live or on TV, or perhaps even if you listen to a radio commentary. You still won't understand everything that's going on, or everything that's said, but any book that tried to get you to that point would be so long, so detailed and so complex that you probably wouldn't have picked it up in the first place!

That said, the important thing is that you now have a foundation to build on, and as you watch and listen, you'll gradually pick up new words and new concepts which will enable you to get even more enjoyment from the game. There's a wealth of material to read too, both in magazine and book form and, of course, in the shape of newspaper articles and reports, and there is obviously much to learn from those quarters.

So where you go from here is up to you – you might even go on to look at one of the books that purport to provide an introduction for the layman but in fact require quite a lot of knowledge to appreciate! What is certain is that the more you know about cricket, the more you'll enjoy it...

About the Author

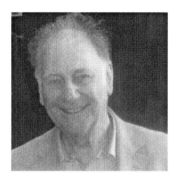

According to his birth certificate, says Tony, he's old - 80 in January 2013 – but he says don't believe it, because he doesn't! He thinks it's a conspiracy to get rid of him – since he lives in Cheltenham, almost certainly GCHQ have something to do with it, and his birth certificate is clearly a forgery...

Although his main career when he was younger was teaching French – in schools, a teacher-training college and a university – he also had a secondary career as an examiner: for more than twenty-five years he was Chief Examiner in French for GCE 'O' Level (and, later, GCSE), and Chief Oral Examiner in French for GCE 'A' Level.

But he has also been a writer for a long time, and has thirty or more French, German and Spanish textbooks to his credit, as well as a history of the Cheltenham Bach Choir (he has been a very enthusiastic choral singer for a long time and, although he has now retired from singing, he is Vice-President of the Cheltenham Bach Choir), and two books on cricket, including this one.

He learned a great deal about cricket when he was a teen-ager, watching many of the greatest players in the history of the game, e.g. Bradman, Hammond, Hutton, Compton, Weekes, Worrall, Walcott, Lindwall, Laker, Trueman, Tyson - to name but a few!

60

In the last year or two he has turned his attention to fiction, and his first novel, *Before the Swallow Dares*, was published in October 2012. His second, called *The Heat of the Kitchen* was published in July 2013, and has been very well received.

Although, as Tony says, he's getting on a bit, he's far from being done with writing. He may not manage to write as many novels as Balzac, the author who was his special subject when he appeared on *Mastermind* four years ago at the age of 76, but he'll give it a go!

If you want to know a bit more about him, have a look at his website: www.tony-whelpton.co.uk. You can also follow him on Twitter: @SwallowDares.

Lightning Source UK Ltd.
Milton Keynes UK
UKOW04f2310260515

252337UK00002B/38/P